Please return to Raise

on your own

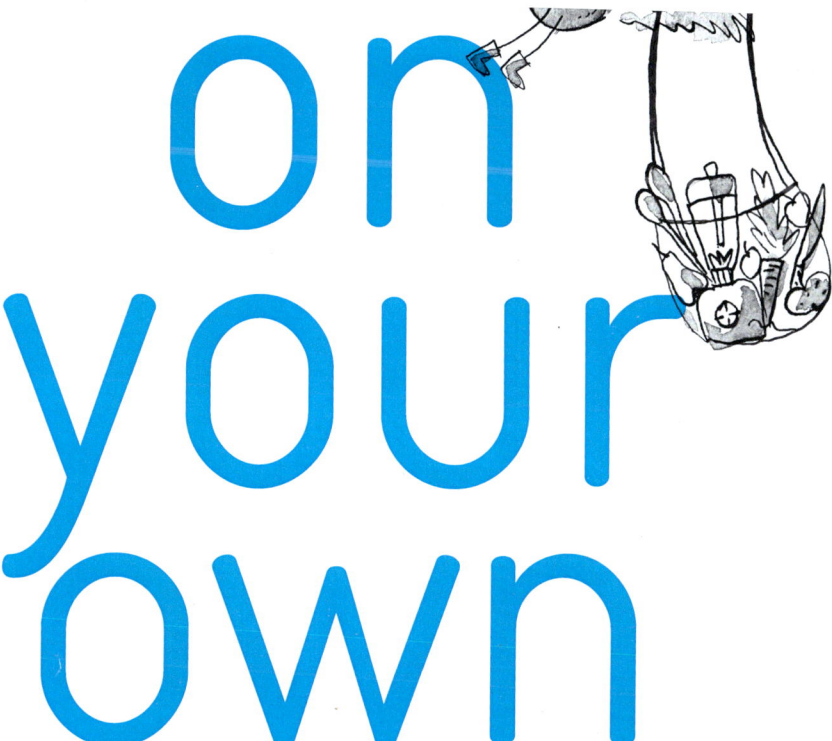

a nutrition and lifestyle recipe for a balanced young adult life

Teresa Fernandez-Gil, Ph.D.

On Your Own: A Nutrition and Lifestyle Recipe for a Balanced Young Adult Life
© 2014 Teresa Fernandez-Gil

Design by Florence Van Acker, drawings by Leila Strebelle.

All rights reserved. No part of this book may be reproduced or transmitted in any form or by any means, electronic or mechanical, including photocopying, recording or by any information storage and retrieval system, without permission in writing from the author. For information, contact **Teresa Fernandez Gil** at **www.teresafernandez-gil.com**

Disclaimer: The content of this book is for general instruction only, and it is not intended to take the place of, or eliminate, the reader's relationship with a physician or other professional.

―――――――――――――

"Health is a state of complete harmony of the body, mind and spirit. When one is free from physical disabilities and mental distractions, the gates of the soul open."
– BKS Iyengar

―――――――――――――

To the infinite possibilities of a young life,
to Alvaro, Pedro, Clara, and Ana Teresa

contents

who am I to give advice? — p.1

fly from the nest and build your own — p.3

welcome to your very own world! — p.5

you only have one body! — p.11

THE PLAN — p.15

1. how it works — p.21
2. the guidelines — p.29
3. getting ready — p.43
4. helpers — p.49
5. recipes and guides — p.55
6. wrapping up at the end of the 3 weeks — p.71

EXTRA ADVICE — p.75

other cares of the self — p.75

other useful concepts — p.81

when out of track — p.82

favorite reading list — p.85

favorite websites — p.87

who am I to give advice?

Well, let me start by telling you that ever since I was a child, I was very sensitive about food and how it made me feel. That's how I began my difficult search for the right way to eat. I knew from the start that this was not going to be an easy journey, and years and years of study made the whole thing even more complicated. The more I learned about human physiology and the chemistry of food, the more complex everything looked.

During my doctorate studies, I spent some time working at one of the top nutrition labs in Cambridge (UK), and I discovered that my colleagues had no clue about how to eat properly to take care of themselves! It literally made me cry. While broadening my approach, I slowly started to realize that I needed to simplify it at the same time. I learned that calories were not all created equal, and that the molecules in food were not all there was to it.

You may be surprised to learn that nutrition is actually a very young science, one that is still trying to build a strong and well-accepted foundation. Some people like to compare it to geography in the Era of Discoveries, when each new finding came from a radical change of direction. Michael Pollan, the best selling food writer, even says, "[Nutrition] is a flawed science that knows much less than it cares to admit."

As a mother, raising four children opened new worlds for me. I realized that we all react in different ways to the food we eat. I had started to understand the importance of bio-individuality when I came across Joshua Rosenthal's eye-opening online program in Integrative Nutrition, the largest nutrition school in the world. My health coaching practice definitely confirmed what I learned from the program, and everything came full circle. After many years of practice, I invite you to share in what I have learned from my studies and my personal family experiences.

Before you begin, I want to start by telling you that this Plan was developed through my own experimentation with different practical teachings. I have been hugely inspired by three main works: *Clean* by Dr. Junger, *Perfect Health* by Dr. Deepak Chopra, and by the Ayurvedic Challenge and other teachings from lifespa.com by Dr. Douillard, my ayurveda guru. After using my own body (and those of my husband and kids, too!) as guinea pigs for years, I have come up with my own approach. I also credit many other inspirational sources that I, as a health counselor, am in touch with day in and day out. I have tested the Plan with many, many patients, and I have continued learning from every outcome. The Plan I propose to you now is thoroughly proven... and it works!

fly from the nest and build your own

My oldest son, Alvaro, has recently left the nest to study abroad. Close friends who have already gone through this change warned us about the feeling of emptiness we are going to experience. Many feel as though he is still young (he's only seventeen!) and are certain that we are going to miss each other terribly. But I, by nature an optimist at heart, have a steady sense of confidence in life. Moreover, I've always felt that our children don't actually belong to us; we look after them in their early years, and then they fly away, out of the nest, towards other destinations and other lives. Despite this undying confidence, and because I am a nutritionist, I struggled with a very strong professional bias, and the only thing I could really think of was, "Will he know how to feed himself well? Will he know how to keep himself strong and healthy?"

For months, I found myself thinking about which appliances would be ideal for him to have in his student dorm for cooking and preparing foods, which products would be indispensable for me to put in his suitcase, and which others should I have delivered later. I often annoyed him with this. After weeks of bothering him with my "very important questions," he finally looked at me and said, "Please, Mom, can you just write everything down, so I can read it when I get there?"

And so, as I did this, I realized that you might also appreciate the wisdom and advice. You might not know it yet, but learning how to take care of yourself properly in order to be vital and healthy is crucial in order to lead a happy and fulfilling life! And while the body and mind may be infinitely complex, the best medicine is usually incredibly simple! The promise of this book is that you are going to learn from the inside out, and this is what I would like to pass on to you.

Starting an independent life as a young adult is a time of intense learning. It is also the first time in your life when you can really make decisions for yourself. Yeah! **I hope that you will use this book to enhance your curiosity about food, digestion, and lifestyle, so you can get the best out of your new life!**

welcome to your very own world!

Congratulations! You're on your own and can now organize your days as you like and be the absolute master of your own lifestyle and diet. What an experience!

It looks like you have decided to take care of your health and lifestyle — what a great idea! Or perhaps someone else is concerned about you, someone who loves you, and decided to give you this book. Whatever the reason, you are reading it, and I hope that you find the information both helpful and interesting. I know you're busy, and I want you to really read this book because it will change your life, which is why I kept it short. I hope you can get through it in one sitting (or two).

Food is one of the basic necessary elements for living a healthy life, and learning about it is an essential step in the path toward independence. Taking responsibility for your own health can seem daunting. Even more so if, like most of us, you found your meals ready and on the table whenever you needed them…because you had a saint of a mother (or father) that took care of all that, had a cafeteria readily available, or maintained a well-stocked freezer with ready-made meals. Or, maybe, you were not very interested in food at all and just grabbed food here and there for fuel.

I'm quite sure that one or more of the following scenarios apply to you. Let's see …

- **"I have a little knowledge but not enough."** Some of you may already know how to cook a little or may feel very much at home in the kitchen, while others haven't so much as touched a saucepan. Perhaps you learned some basic nutrition as part of your high school studies, but, surely, this was a little too theoretical and lacking in practical applications.

- **"Sometimes I eat for emotional reasons."** Most people think of eating as a pleasure or as a means to fill the emptiness in the stomach, while many others see food as a way to fill other voids that are much harder to identify.

- **"I'm interested in environmental issues, but I don't know how food choices relate to it."** Many of you are conscious of and care about the environment, but perhaps you've never made the connection between the latter and the food that you eat. Fair trade practices, limiting overconsumption and waste, and reducing hunger in the world are concepts that may interest you, and the Plan will help you understand how to connect food choices to these important issues.

- **"I want to be 'healthy,' but I don't know which foods really make a difference."** These days it is 'en vogue' to cultivate one's health. Being healthy, active, fit, and attractive is certainly a must for anyone. Extra pounds, skin impurities, and lack of energy are just a few of the things you would probably be glad to get rid of – if only you knew how.

Wherever you are coming from, and whichever impact you want to make in your life, there is one common way to do it: you just need to learn how to take care of your body and how to choose what you put in it because the foods you select are directly connected to:

- your metabolism and the way you feel physically and emotionally.
- the way you look.
- your focus and mental clarity.
- your energy and ability to work out.
- your health and the prevention of disease.

These food choices also impact:

- the environment and climate change.
- the quality of the water.
- the hunger in the world.
- the work conditions of farmers and distributors in foreign countries.

benefits for you and the planet

When you eat better, you feel better about yourself, are more energetic, and improve your digestion. Your skin becomes brighter and fresher. Your mind also becomes clearer and more active, and your moods are more stable.

The effects on the planet are harder to quantify in the short-term. But any farmer will tell you that a diet that consists mainly of unprocessed, local and seasonal plant food will require less land and water, will generate less waste, emit fewer greenhouse gases, and diminish energy consumption, not to mention sparing much animal suffering. The act of eating is the most intimate encounter that we may have with our planet: what we eat becomes a part of us. Without the nutrients that Nature supplies, we would, of course, not survive. It is time to redevelop a nurturing relationship with Her. What we eat and how we care for ourselves affects how we relate to the environmental issues on the planet. Therefore, it is really important to take some time at every meal to reflect on the food you are about to eat. Think about how it arrived on your plate. Who contributed to its production, transport, and commercialization? And ask yourself if it is in its natural form or has been transformed in some way.

life! be fit for it!

Youth makes us think we are immortal, which is an intoxicating feeling. But during this phase, most of us do not realize how fragile our bodies actually are. To stay balanced, we need to pay attention to all the different elements that keep our body functioning well: water, exercise, fresh air, sunshine, sleep, relaxation, and good nutrition.

It's important to rethink the way you eat. Consider this: **eat to live; don't live to eat.** When choosing foods, make sure that you select them for their nourishing power and their ability to digest easily. Occasionally, you will be tempted by items that are readily available or are easy to prepare. Clever marketing even plays a role in your food selection, but try to focus on eating foods that are really good for you instead.

does anyone really know how to eat?

You are probably thinking, "There are fad diets, contradictory nutrition articles in magazines, blogs, and newspapers, health claims on food labels, and assorted advocates of this and that. Is there really a right answer when it comes to eating?"

How does one learn how to feed oneself? Is it intellectual? Should it be taught in school? Is it important to know the rules and facts by heart? Ugh!

It shouldn't be that difficult: wild animals do it just right, and they don't even know how to read! But how do they do it without a scale and a list of ingredients... or without counting calories? How do they manage?

trusting your gut

I am convinced that learning how to take care of your nutrition needs to be done, very literally, from the gut. The only way to actually know what's good for you is to learn by trying something and seeing what your body has to say about it. When using this approach, you get more and more skilled in the art of decoding your body's own signals.

This is exactly what we are going to do here. The promise of this book is that, in just 3 weeks, you'll learn how to nourish yourself and to feel better than ever, in a way that you'll develop using your intuition, thus becoming nutritionally independent. Once you put the Plan into motion, you'll always know what to choose, when to eat it, and how to treat your body, so you'll be free from mood swings, guilt, diet plans, cravings, and exhaustion. The result? Feeling great and being able to use your energy for great things.

I invite you to take this opportunity to develop your intuition. You'll realize that there is no need to rationalize your choices, and that the best key to your health is understanding your individual needs. When you remain attentive to your body's signs, such as digestive reactions, skin blemishes, fat accumulation, and lack of energy ... this will greatly help you choose what to eat. It is important, though, to know that your body knows best when it comes to choosing and dealing with natural food.

Since we all react in different ways to different foods, it can be quite challenging to cook for a family. I know what I am talking about because I raised four kids (plus a husband) that knew about their needs! So, enjoy this independent time and focus on your own needs, desires, and reactions to foods and others ... and learn to listen, to experiment, and to know yourself.

eating healthy is about more than weight

Food that is good for you is not only the kind that makes you lose weight! While lean people do tend to live longer and are statistically sick less often, caring for your waistline is not the main objective behind good nutrition — not at any price! You are probably aware that many diets have been shown to be quite harmful. What is true, however, is that a healthy diet will help you find your ideal weight. It will also improve your overall health!

you only have one body!

During your 20s and 30s, your body is incredibly forgiving, so thinking about the importance of laying a healthy foundation for midlife may be far from your mind. This book is meant to open your eyes to the fact that if you don't do this now, you'll pay the price. I also want you to experience how interesting it can be to take good care of yourself: it is a new world, and you won't be sorry you came to it!

the body and how it works – or doesn't

You know by now that your diet and lifestyle choices will either help or harm the delicate balance at work in a healthy human body. Let's review how the wonderful machine of your body works!

your filtration system

In order to perform all of its different tasks, the human body must take in oxygen, water, and food. Once those have reached the cells, each one, in its own particular way, is used and then transformed into a waste product. Your body has three main organs that act as filters for the metabolic residue of the cellular system: your lungs, kidneys, and liver. They filter huge quantities of waste nonstop every single day (without you ever even thinking about them)! While you probably change your car filters every so often, when was the last time you heard of a lung or liver change? Never ... but your bodily filters need to be protected because you are going to need them for a long and healthy life!

today's habits have consequences

Metabolic waste products, such as CO_2, urea, and cholesterol, are acidic, and when not discarded optimally, they increase our bodies' acidity. This happens when the filters get clogged. Acidity is bad for the system, but do you know what else can contribute to an abnormal increase in acidity? Bad nutrition, insufficient oxygenation, lack of exercise, insufficient hydration, stress, and, of course, toxic habits like alcohol and cigarettes (just to name a few)!

When those waste products stagnate, they hang around in the lymphatic system, which is the body's self-cleaning system, making it thick and sluggish. This, in turn, prevents the cells from absorbing good nutrition and hydration and makes them suffocate in their own waste. Cells may react in different ways to this situation causing different degrees of disease:

Either they just die: This creates different types of situations regarding the tissue in which they are located: Parkinson's and Alzheimer's if in the brain, sclerosis if in the nerves, arthritis if in the joints, and different types of fibrosis in other tissues, such as the ovaries, lungs, and liver...

Or they try to survive by:

- retaining water, which creates swelling, inflammation, and weight gain.
- reducing acidic products into salts by using our skeletal minerals. This creates osteoporosis in the bones and calcifications in the soft tissues. Does this ring a bell?
- draining acids toward the skin, causing dermatitis or psoriasis, or the mucosa, resulting in mouth ulcers, colitis, etc.
- mutating and giving birth to cancerous cells!

lifelong benefits from a lesson learned now

Through these pages, I would like you to learn how to prevent all of this through diet and lifestyle. Now, isn't that cool? Imagine the extra energy you may be able to put toward positive projects instead of fighting against disease. Imagine the huge savings on health insurance!

More and more, a new generation of doctors has started to say that conventional medicine is failing us…especially when it comes to preventive medicine. Twenty-first-century medicine remains focused on treating symptoms for most preventable problems. There is so much more to health than the absence of disease. Meditation, yoga, massage, and nutritional approaches are increasingly embraced as mainstream tools for healing. Prevention is much cheaper than treatment. Preserving balance can ensure an ideal state of health.

When given half a chance, the human body tends to repair itself and regenerate. Once we know all of this, who is going to choose to go through treatment, mainly symptomatic treatment, with its nuisances and side effects, when a change in lifestyle can bring health and vitality? Let's see how!

THE PLAN

By now, I hope you are convinced that the way you take care of your body, and more particularly the way you eat, has a tremendous impact on your life. If you are, you probably want to acquire the knowledge to achieve that healthy state. But you must be wondering why there are so many unhealthy and overweight people out there at a time when most people have a theory about how to be lean and healthy. At a time when, in most countries, packaged foods need to have every ingredient and every nutritional fact clearly written on them. When almost everybody knows plenty of health tricks. So…what's up? How come all this hasn't worked?

Never before has there been so much discussion about health and diet, and in this hyper-informed era of the Internet, tons of information is available for anyone wanting to gain nutritional knowledge. People around the globe are turning to the Internet to research topics concerning their health. They are starting to realize that they need to take care of their health, and that it is no longer a matter of going to the doctor every now and then and praying for good exam results. People nowadays tend to know a lot. So why does this knowledge stay at the theory level instead of producing the desired results (i.e., more healthy bodies)?

knowledge doesn't translate to the plate

In the years that I have been providing nutrition consultations, it has become quite clear to me that it is difficult to translate theories and facts onto a dinner plate. Even when you read all the information on the labels and use an app that calculates the totals, how can you be sure of your magnesium consumption on a given day? What about the level of calcification in your bones? Or the rate at which you absorb different nutrients? Tricky, huh? It would be difficult to know all this even if you worked at a laboratory.

you don't need willpower – you need to know your body

And then, what about cravings? Almost everyone is aware of the fact that eating a whole pint of ice cream just before going to bed is not the best idea, but...have you met many people who can fight those late-night cravings just by knowing when and when not to eat ice cream? I think most people have plenty of willpower. What they tend to lack is the awareness of how they're being affected by what they eat, the necessary knowledge in order to make changes, and the belief that change is possible. What if instead of getting more willpower, you focused on gaining a deeper understanding of your body and the way it responds to the food you eat?

let your body be your guide

All of this has left me and other people thinking that rationalization doesn't seem to go well with nutrition. Too much thinking is actually a bad idea for your health. These things need to be learned from the inside out, and that is how the idea of the program and the Plan emerged. People need guidance. They need to experiment, analyze, and then draw their own conclusions. They don't need intellectual knowledge as much as they need to know their own bodies, so they can decode their signs better. Because, you know what? They do have a laboratory: their own bodies. And when carefully listened to, they give us all the answers we need.

This Plan will help you learn more about the best nutrition sources available, the most effective way to consume them in order to convert them into premium fuel, and how to listen to your body in order to get to know which foods and practices are best suited to your particular self. This is a proven way to learn what is good for you. It is a simple, straightforward strategy. I want to liberate you from having to count food calories or grams. This is not a diet. It is a way of life.

The closer you stick to the guidelines, the faster you will see results, and the more clearly you will recognize your body's reactions. I don't want you to become a food freak; on the contrary, the goal is that this way of eating will become second nature. You just need to take the initial plunge and experience the effects…and 3 weeks seems to do the trick.

eating naturally and instinctively

We have seen in the wild that animals get their nutrition just right without thinking about it. They achieve perfect bodies, shiny hair, and great elegance…without giving a thought to it. Looks like Mother Nature, our one and only master, has had a perfect plan all along. She provides her creatures with all the knowledge they need for a fulfilling life. Nature has always been there for us, too, but most of us have been ignoring Her. Nothing in nature, except humans, needs a brain in order to get proper nutrition. Animals are instinctive; their gut tells them what to eat. Shouldn't we try listening a bit more and getting in touch with our animal nature?

"Nature is the source of all true knowledge. She has her own logic, her own laws; she has no effect without cause, no invention without necessity."
– Leonardo DaVinci

Don't fight Mother Nature. Live in harmony with Her. Watch the daily cycles, the seasons, and the signs in your body. When we eat what She offers us, our bodies can function in a natural way, and their reactions may guide us the way Nature intended. So... eating natural food to understand our natural reaction is the main principle of our Plan.

CHAPTER 1

how it works

why the plan

As Dr. Mark Hyman, one of the pioneering doctors on functional medicine, puts it, "If you eat crap, you feel like crap." The best way to get out from under this "crap" circle is by following an appropriate regimen long enough so that you start feeling marvelous, so marvelous that you want to keep that feeling at almost any price. I have been sharing this **KEEP IN-KEEP OUT** diet with my patients long enough to know that 98 percent of them have had tremendous improvements in health and energy levels (the other 2 percent were probably cheating!). By **KEEP IN-KEEP OUT**, I mean a diet that eliminates all foods that usually induce irritation, toxicity, and/or inflammation, in order to help your body recognize its signals. They help you learn what to eat in order to thrive and what to avoid because it doesn't serve you.

Some people think that following a restrictive diet is extreme...but let me tell you what I think is extreme: taking pills with horrendous side effects; having surgery (although we are all glad it exists when we really need it); chemotherapy and radiotherapy; and even taking painkillers is more extreme than a restrictive diet.

A KEEP IN-KEEP OUT diet is the best way to tap into your intuition. It's like pressing your body's reset button. It decreases inflammation, cleanses your lymphatic system, provokes mental clarity, and rejuvenates your digestive tract. And among other wonderful perks, it creates the shortest path to increased bodily awareness. Remember, we are working on your bio-individuality here. It is about finding what works best for you, then creating your own diet and daily routine based on your individual desires and needs.

pick your approach

- **"I need to know more before jumping in."** Perhaps you need to know exactly what you are getting into or need more convincing before starting. Maybe you want to learn about food and lifestyle but know it isn't practical to start the Plan at this moment. If so, then continue reading the book from beginning to end. You may want to start introducing changes gradually instead of jumping into the Plan. Try experimenting with smoothies then transition to the 3-meal-a-day pattern, etc. You can then launch the Plan when you are absolutely ready.

- **"I'm ready now."** Maybe you like to learn by doing or don't want to spend time reading now. That's fine, too. Just skip the 'why' and the 'how' in the next two sections and go directly to the 'guidelines' chapter and plunge into the Plan. You can always do the reading afterwards.

reduce inflammation naturally

Inflammation is the body's natural reaction to some kind of stress. It is supposed to be an instant reaction, not turned on for prolonged periods of time. But this is what is currently happening to millions of people. If the body is constantly under assault and exposed to irritants, the inflammation response stays on.

And we have created this problem. Our society is "inflamed" because the foods we grow are unbalanced and also "inflamed." For example, farmed fish are fed with food they would never choose if they had a voice; cows eat corn and soy while static in their boxes instead of grazing green pastures; vegetables are grown in poor soils with unnatural fertilizers; and crops are hybridized and genetically modified (GMO). In the case of this already "inflamed" produce, it is often further denatured by lack of freshness and processing, including the addition of preservatives and additives.

A diet rich in processed carbohydrates and bad quality fats is pro-inflammatory. When we ingest these so-called "foods," our body reacts by creating inflammation. This translates into that hard-to-identify body malaise and cloudiness of mind. You know that you are inflamed when you have headaches, aching or swollen joints, red or congested tissues, skin rashes, or are suffering from asthma, coronary artery disease, or even Alzheimer's and Parkinson's.

By eliminating irritants, toxic molecules, and inflammation triggers like sugar, dairy, gluten, and all the other elements in the KEEP OUT portion of the Plan, you will not only reduce inflammation but also have more energy available to aid in the process of detoxification. By consuming fresh, mostly plant-based, unprocessed natural food, rich in antioxidants and healthy fats for 3 weeks, you will reduce most of the inflammation, and your system will be clean enough to be able to identify a denatured product when it enters your system again. You'll have reset the natural system that is your health. Reducing stress, thanks to some of the elements in your daily routine, will help reduce inflammation, too.

choose food instinctively

Natural fresh seasonal produce comes packed with all the elements needed for its digestion and absorption. This food awakens your body to the right signals, so you can easily detect when to stop eating or when to have more. A 3-week program with real fresh food and a conducive lifestyle are what the body needs to start working optimally and to send the signals that are going to guide you toward making choices that are right for you. You will finally have a balanced diet guided by your own instincts instead of one that turns nutrition into an intellectual headache.

watch out for these monsters

- foods that are too sugary, too salty, or full of engineered fats.
- processed foods, which lose all or part of their minerals, vitamins, fiber, and natural fat along the way.
- foods that have been overcooked, radiated, or even microwaved.

All these unnatural concoctions can disrupt your metabolism and bodily functions and leave you with a hard to identify uneasiness.

eat three meals and burn more fat

At some time, everyone has followed a six (or even eight!) meal daily plan. It was a fad in dietetics based on the fact that most of us have a disrupted glycemic metabolism, which means that our glucose levels go up and down, uncontrolled, all day long. Experts believed that eating several snacks a day could tame this pattern. The truth is that if you have a diet that achieves glucose balance, you will feel more energized because the exhausting efforts your body goes through when attempting to control glucose levels will cease, and you'll find you don't need snacks. Particularly because you will also be free from the cravings that this rollercoaster creates.

At the same time, you'll start burning fat during the fasting periods that this diet provides. You are probably wondering how all of this magic is going to happen. It is quite simple, really. You will be very close to accomplishing all of this just by starting off the day with a perfectly balanced meal. Take a look at the recipes in the breakfast section. All these options are designed to maintain glucose and insulin levels at a normal range. This means your cravings and mid-morning energy slump will all but disappear, which will help you reach your lunchtime energized and relaxed (while burning fat in your body).

Lunch will then become a leisurely meal, not one influenced by hypoglycemia (and you won't find yourself gorging on bread and butter while waiting for your meal to be served). You'll be in complete control and will again be able to choose the perfect blend of ingredients to keep that blissful state all the way to dinner (and, again, still burning fat). Without the up and down glucose levels, fat is a fuel that burns steadily.

Most people, during their high school and college years, spend their days feeling lethargic. Ring any bells? When you experience this new glucose-stable state, you will never ever want to go back to that rollercoaster! It is the same sensation as when you felt satin or cashmere for the first time. Once you've felt something that good, how could you even think of wearing itchy wool again?

Just try it for 3 weeks, and you will see. And you will be astonished by how little food you actually need. After you make the initial investment in superfoods and other materials, you'll see your food expenses go down as well!

eliminate toxic buildup

A perfect functioning body is also one that detoxifies on a daily basis. You have probably stored excess toxins from your not-so-clean routines from the past, and unfortunately, there are going to be plenty of others entering your system every day. And this is going to happen, I'm sad to say, even if you have the cleanest diet because there are so many things that you can't control, such as environmentally toxic products, furniture and carpeting chemicals, cleaning products, and even cosmetics, to name just a few. So, at the same time that you try to reduce toxins, you are going to learn how to best help your body get rid of most of them.

The fasting periods between meals allow for the melting of stored fat. Fat-soluble toxins are then released, which can circulate in the now well-hydrated lymphatic system and be neutralized in the liver and gallbladder. They need to be discarded along with their mucus coating. Hydration, fiber and quality fat will help you achieve this wonderful process.

By following the Plan, you'll also increase elimination through the already existing elimination channels of your body: good daily bowel movements, rehydration, skin brushing, tongue scraping, and deep breathing.

preserve alkalinity and help the lymphatic system

The balance between alkalinity and acidity in our internal chemistry is vital. The body must be in a balanced alkaline state to operate at its best, but the by-products of much of its functions are acidic. So, we need to pay attention to help our bodies deal with those by-products and still stay alkaline. Pollutants, physical and physiological stress, and toxins all push our bodies toward acidity. Clear signs of acidity are puffy eyes, fragile nails and hair, and a porous non-taut face. Pain in the soles of your feet when you first step on the floor in the morning and recurrent infections are also other signs.

The body has, of course, its mechanisms to neutralize the acidity by combining the acids with minerals (sodium, potassium, calcium, and magnesium). These minerals then become an essential part of your diet. But beware: non-organic, processed foods often lack these essential minerals. A healthy alkaline body is best supported by a healthy alkaline lifestyle: good food choices full of mineral-rich ingredients, exercise, deep breathing, and salt bathing all support alkalinity by pumping up the lymphatic system, so it will eliminate acids and toxins.

improve digestion

A body that functions well is a body that digests optimally. You know that your digestion is good when you have a daily bowel movement within two hours of waking up, have no acid reflux or mucus in your stools, and can digest a fatty healthy meal without feeling heavy, bloated, or uncomfortable. To be a good detoxifier, you need to be a good digester. Given the right conditions, your digestive system will regain strength and perform its functions with ease.

Here's a fun fact: 90 percent of the cells in your body are not yours. Huh? Actually, they belong to the wonderful 'bugs' that colonize your body, particularly your bowels. You understand why it is so important to keep those guys happy, don't you? The best way to do this is to remove the irritants in your body by adding the right amount of good fats, fiber, and natural probiotics. You'll learn more about this in the recipe and guide sections of the book.

understand your body and its reactions

When well tuned, your body is the world's best laboratory. During the 3-week Plan, you will gradually see your energy levels soar, your sleep and moods improve, your digestion strengthen, and your skin glow! When resuming old, unhealthy habits during and after the reintroduction days, your body will tell you very clearly which ones are okay once in a while, and which ones are a no-no.

CHAPTER 2

the guidelines

for three weeks, you will be having:
- **three meals a day. NO SNACKS!** There are no restrictions regarding the quantity you eat at a meal. At first, you want to make sure you'll have enough to carry you until the next meal. Gradually, when the glucose highs disappear, you will auto-regulate, I promise!
- **a restrictive, restorative diet.** No sugar, no dairy, no gluten… choose your ingredients from the nourishing and delicious KEEP-IN list.
- **lots of water.**
- **a daily alkalinizing routine.**

remember

- The fresher the foods, the more potent their nutrients.
- Local, seasonal, and organic ingredients are preferable whenever available – for obvious reasons.
- The more nutritious your meals, the more successful your 3-meal-per-day plan will be. This will turn on your feel-good fat metabolism.

ingredients

KEEP IN	KEEP OUT
fruits and vegetables: all fresh and in season fruits and vegetables, including seaweed	**CORN**
vegetable milk: rice milk, almond milk, oat milk, hemp milk, and coconut milk	**DAIRY:** milk, cheese, cream, yogurt, butter, ice cream, and soy milk
non gluten grains: rice, quinoa, millet, amaranth, buckwheat, oats	**GLUTEN:** wheat, spelt, kamut, rye
animal protein: the cleanest meat, fish, poultry, and eggs possible (pasture raised, free-range, organic, wild...)	bacon, cold cuts, and sausage; non-organic beef, veal, chicken, pork, or farmed fish (do as best you can)
vegetable protein: lentils, all kinds of beans, chickpeas	**SOY** beans and soy bean products
nuts and seeds: almonds, walnuts, hazelnuts, pistachios, and pine nuts. Hemp, sesame, pumpkin, and sunflower seeds. All nut and seed butters	Peanuts and peanut butter
oils: cold-pressed olive oil, sesame oil, and coconut oil	margarine, butter, mayonnaise, and all seed oils (except sesame)
drinks: filtered or mineral water. Green, white, and herbal teas	Alcohol, coffee, caffeinated beverages, soft drinks, and fruit juice
sweeteners: whole fresh fruit, dried fruit	**SUGAR**, maple syrup, all artificial sweeteners...
condiments: sea salt, vinegar, all herbs and spices, wheat-free Tamari (traditionally prepared fermented soy sauce)	refined salt, sugar added-balsamic vinegar, ketchup, soy sauce, teriyaki...

how to choose your food

What a big question! Let me share with you a few principles that guide my choices.

— whole, natural foods —

You want to choose your foods as close to their natural state as possible. Wild would be ideal, of course, but wouldn't be easy to get, so try to choose well-grown food from healthy soils. This means choosing organic foods or items from a reliable source that is certified (and one that you trust).

When you eat animals, it is very important to know how those animals have been treated and what they have been fed. Look for wild, pasture-raised, or free-range items. Very soon, you will develop a sense for the wonderful qualities of these well-raised products. Your palate will detect the higher fat quality of a wild fish, and your eyes will perceive the darker yellow of butter or egg yolks from animals raised on grass instead of grains.

Industrial processing strips food of many of its nutrients. It also generally involves adding preservatives, colors, flavors, sweeteners, or lots of salt. Don't get fooled by the words "fortified" or "enriched" on bread or cereal labels. It doesn't make sense to remove nutrients in the first part of the process and then add chemical versions at the end. Natural foods work beautifully and are more complex than any laboratory can create.

— seasonal —

In spring, green grass sprouts everywhere. Cows can go back to grazing fields and producing the best milk of the year. Leafy greens and berries are in season. The hens lay their best eggs.

In summer, nature is generous. There is a festival of fruits and fruit-vegetables, such as tomatoes, cucumbers, peppers, zucchini, eggplant, and more.

Fall brings grains, nuts and seeds, and root vegetables... all energetic products that can be stored because winter, in most places, has little to offer. Traditionally, people relied on stored preserves and animal food during winter. Our ancestors ate seasonally because they didn't have any other choice.

There are two reasons that you should follow the seasons. First: freshness. If you eat what is in season where you live, you'll find well-ripened fruits and vegetables that have had shorter transport and storage times. Secondly, when you live in harmony with nature, you'll see that you crave what the season is about to offer you. Spring's greens and berries are detoxifiers after a winter season of excess. Sun-filled fruits and veggies meet our increased demand for energy on long active summer days. And grains, seeds, and nuts are all rich in nutrients, which build insulation and protection for the colder months of the year.

SPRING
leafy greens and berries

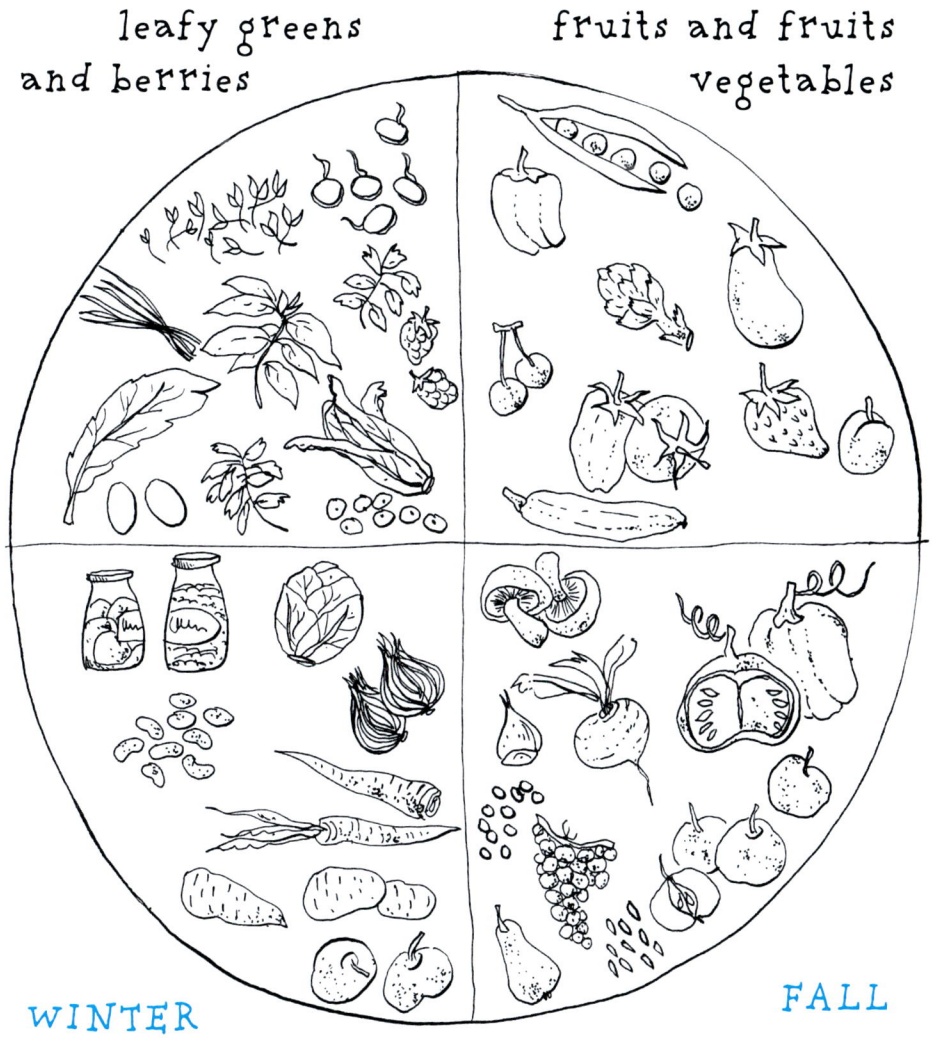

SUMMER
fruits and fruits vegetables

WINTER
stored preserves, grains, nuts and vegetables from the fall

FALL
root vegetables, grains and nuts, fruits and mushrooms

— sustainable —

Choosing a diet that is rich in environmentally friendly plant products is already a very positive choice. Organic farming is more sustainable because it preserves the soil, so your food choices not only have an impact on your health but that of the planet, too.

The production of food requires energy, water, fertilization, machinery, transportation, and human resources to name just a few. What, how, where, and when it is produced has a huge impact on the environment and the people that work directly or indirectly in that area. When you eat seasonal, local, fresh vegetables that you buy from the grower at a farmer's market, for instance, your impact on the planet is small. It can become even smaller if you plant your own vegetable garden.

Some food industries, especially industrial meat production, are known for wasting resources and polluting the water. Fish is also problematic since the natural resources are shrinking, and the industrial production pollutes the environment and requires a great deal of natural resources. For example, farmed fish are fed prepared flour, which is made from small ocean fish. The amount of fish required to make this flour exceeds the number of fish it will feed, and this leads to overfishing. This doesn't mean that you need to become a vegetarian. But if you are particularly picky about the quality of your animal protein, it will directly reduce your consumption.

— traditional —

People eating according to the rules of a traditional food culture, such as Mediterranean, Japanese, rural Chinese, etc., are generally much healthier than people eating a contemporary Western diet. Several decades ago, our markets and supermarkets were not as diversified as they are today.

In the Spain of my childhood, it was impossible to find mangoes or avocados, but endless aisles of processed carbohydrates, such as cereal, biscuits, and bread, as well as chemically extracted oils, processed sauces, and poor-quality soy and dairy didn't exist either. While we have multiplied our options, we have lost part of our traditional eating culture at the same time, at least in the example of Spain that I know so well.

When making food choices, you may choose to stick to your own tradition or adopt another that has stood the test of time, or, maybe, blend all of them as I personally do.

let's take a natural food tour!
— vegetables are priority #1 —

These are the foods that need the least transformation before arriving on your plate. Varied, colorful, attractive – they can be eaten raw, blended, juiced, or gently cooked. They have a whole array of interesting nutrients: antioxidants, vitamins, minerals, good fats, and, last but not least, fiber.

- **green, leafy vegetables** (kale, Swiss chard, spinach, endive, arugula, radicchio, lettuce, watercress, dandelion, parsley, coriander, basil, etc.) are rich in chlorophyll, the only molecule on Earth able to transform inorganic matter into organic matter. They are an undeniable source of life and should be given absolute priority. Plus, the beneficial bacteria in your gut loves them!

- **flower vegetables** are the edible blossoms of cruciferous plants (cabbage, cauliflower, broccoli, sauerkraut, etc.). They protect against degenerative diseases and should be on your plate at least once a day.

- **root vegetables** (carrots, potatoes, beets, sweet potatoes, and onions) **and fruit vegetables** (squash, zucchini, pumpkins, and also tomatoes, peppers, cucumbers, eggplant, etc.) are often sweet and colorful, and they make an excellent alternative for bad carbs.

- **beans or pulses (legumes)** are a source of protein and lots of other interesting elements (lentils, all types of beans, and chickpeas). They are best consumed in small quantities, preferably sprouted, which makes them more digestible and nutritious. Beware of bad quality soy products, like soy milk, soy yogurt, and other soy products that have not been properly fermented.

- **seaweed** and other sea vegetables (nori, dulce, wakame, arame, kombu, etc.) are also delicious and nutritious and should be part of your regular diet.

— don't be afraid of fats, but be choosy —

Healthy fat is an essential component of food that you definitely need to put back in your diet if you haven't cared about it lately or have been afraid of it. Fat is back. Yeah! Indispensable for strengthening cells, most particularly, brain cells, fat also lubricates joints, insulates the body, binds toxins from the liver, maintains healthy cholesterol levels in your blood and brain, and provides energy.

- **oils.** Choose cold-pressed oils from fruit, particularly olive oil and coconut oil. Together with sesame oil, they have been used for centuries and haven't ever been linked to health problems. You should avoid other seed oils altogether. Their processing and tendency to turn rancid make them unsuitable for human consumption.

- raw **nuts and seeds**, nut and seed butters.

- **fatty fruits.** Olives, coconuts, and especially avocados, which are one of the world's most perfect foods.

- fat wild **fish** from cold waters should not to be forgotten either.

- **dairy.** Butter is a nutritious and delicious food if it is organic, comes from pasture-raised cows, and is made, preferably, from raw milk. Its purified form, ghee, has nothing but the best elements of the dairy family. Remember, dairy is restricted during the 3-week Plan, but you can add it back afterwards.

And remember: fat doesn't make you fat. The farmers fatten their animals with grain, not fat!

— whole grains and other carbs —

Whole grains are very comforting and filling, and their production causes much less pollution than meat production. Always choose whole and gluten-free varieties and combine them with a sizable amount of vegetables.

- rice
- oats
- buckwheat
- millet
- amaranth
- non-grain carbs, such as potatoes and quinoa

Gluten is a well-known inflammatory food and bowel irritant, very probably both, because we are overexposed to it, and because the production of the foods that contain it is highly industrialized. Most people feel genuine relief when avoiding it. Feel it for yourself with the KEEP IN-KEEP OUT program!

— quality **proteins** are important —

Among the natural foods available to us, there are proteins from two main sources: animal and vegetable.

- **animal proteins** are found in meat, fish, eggs, and dairy products.
- **vegetable proteins** come mainly from legumes and can also be found in grains, seeds, and nuts, but in smaller proportions.

Animal products are rich in urea and uric acid, and at the end of the food chain, they are more concentrated in synthetic toxins (antibiotics, hormones, and pesticides) than plant products. They generate acidity and mucus in your body and increase cortisol levels (the stress hormone). You've already learned that producing them causes pollution, but this does not mean that you must remove them from your diet.

Consume various animal proteins in small quantities. Choose different kinds of meat, fish, and eggs, and think of legumes as a nice nourishing alternative. Treat yourself to the best possible affordable quality products: fresh, organic, wild, and pasture-raised. Only eat animals that have been well taken care of or those that are wild. For fish, small is usually better because it is usually cleaner.

Dairy products have also become problematic because of their hyper-industrialization and their over-consumption. One thing is certain, they are not as calcifying as originally believed (and there are more women with osteoporosis in France than in any country in Africa). If you decide to keep dairy products in your diet after the 3-week Plan, choose the highest quality from the freshest source.

— fruits —

Fruits bring a touch of freshness and sweetness to your meals. They are both nourishing and cleansing and should be consumed only when in season (although bananas, mangos, and frozen berries are some of the indulgences that I allow myself). When well combined, you'll learn how to do this in the recipe section, they are a highly enjoyable part of your diet.

— spoil yourself with good condiments —

- opt for **fresh herbs,** such as basil, coriander, parsley, oregano, chives, and rosemary, especially organically grown varieties. You can grow most of them on your windowsill almost year round.

- the quality of the **salt** you use is essential: unrefined sea salt, Himalayan salt, Celtic salt, and "fleur de sel," are good choices. Tamari soy is used in Asia, and when produced in a traditional way (the soy needs to be fermented), it is a great asset to your kitchen.

- **spices,** such as ginger, cinnamon, cayenne pepper, paprika, turmeric, and dried aromatic herbs are welcome and will provide zest and color to your recipes. They are excellent sources of antioxidants and have many other qualities: anti-inflammatory, anti-infective, and anti-cancerous. Everyone is talking about turmeric these days, and it has been in the news for very good reasons. When combined with black pepper, its power is greatly increased. Cayenne is also a darling of good nutrition because it eases digestion.

— superfoods —

While each food listed below belongs in one of the earlier groups, I'd like to emphasize their importance here because they are going to be some of your greatest helpers as you adapt to your new routine and beyond. Experts call them "super" because of their nutrient density and minimal waste. They are packed with antioxidants, vitamins, and minerals, and are easy to store and take along on your trips. Since you can carry them with you and add them to the meals you eat away from home, you can always enjoy good nutrition. They can be quite expensive, but they are so nutritionally dense (no losses, everything is used) that their cost per serving isn't high.

- **the berries:** goji berries, mulberries, and açai
- **the seeds:** hemp seeds, flax seeds, and chia seeds
- **the greens:** spirulina, chlorella, and wheatgrass
- and, of course, **raw cacao** and maca powder

— fermented food —

This next food group sounds complicated, but it really isn't. When foods, like pickles, are preserved, they go through a natural process called lacto-fermentation. During the process, natural lactobacilli, as well as other beneficial strains of bacteria, grow and produce lots of lactic acid. The lactic acid preserves the food while slowly releasing sugars from the cellulose to feed the good bacteria, which your body depends upon. Fruits, vegetables, and dairy products that are fermented in this way increase the number of 'good bugs' in the body. The foods become natural probiotics and promote a healthy, robust immune system. They should be used particularly during the winter months.

- kefir and kombucha
- traditionally prepared pickles
- natural sauerkraut

— drinks —

Water, water, and water. And then herbal teas and lightly steeped green or white tea. During the 3-week Plan, you won't be able to have fruit juice because it wreaks havoc on your sugar metabolism. Freshly squeezed green juices can be interesting and helpful when fasting or detoxing but not during our Plan. Coffee interferes with your metabolism, increases stress, and interferes with restful sleep. If your caffeine intake is under control, you may want to keep the after lunch coffee but try to be picky about the quality. Alcohol can also be a great disruptor and a sure source of sugar. You may want to try 3 weeks without it and then reintroduce just one glass of very good wine during a meal.

CHAPTER 3

getting ready

You want to start by taking some time to make up your mind, carefully **choose your start date**, and get prepared. Look very carefully at your calendar to maximize your chances of success. You don't want to start your 3-week Plan during the winter holidays, during a stressful time, or when travelling with family or friends. You want to choose a date that will allow you to have one whole week when you are totally under control. At the beginning of the second week, most things start becoming second nature, and you'll be able to better handle difficult situations.

I highly recommend that you **keep a journal** in which you record the experiences you are going through. You can include goals, recipes, body signs, reactions, and feelings. Your journal will become an interesting document, which you may want to consult on different occasions (i.e., before going to the doctor or your health coach, or before you begin the 3-week Plan again, etc.). Setting a fixed time to write, perhaps after dinner, works best.

Start **organizing your material.**

In your kitchen, you are going to need:

- **knives** and **chopping boards**

- **a blender.** It will be extremely useful when preparing smoothies, soups, dips, and nut butters, although it is not absolutely necessary. You can certainly follow your 3-week Plan without soups or smoothies, but if you decide to shop for one (with the money you are going to save by eliminating Starbucks for 21 days!), review your budget and available kitchen space and then check out the models available. With a blender, you really get what you pay for, so focus on the power of the motor and the quality of the blades. For around $100, I recommend an immersion hand blender or single serve blender like the NutriBullet, which is extremely useful if you are in a college dorm or small apartment. If you are like me, and intend to use your blender more often than your toothbrush (and can also spend a little bit more), then a high speed Vitamix is what you want.

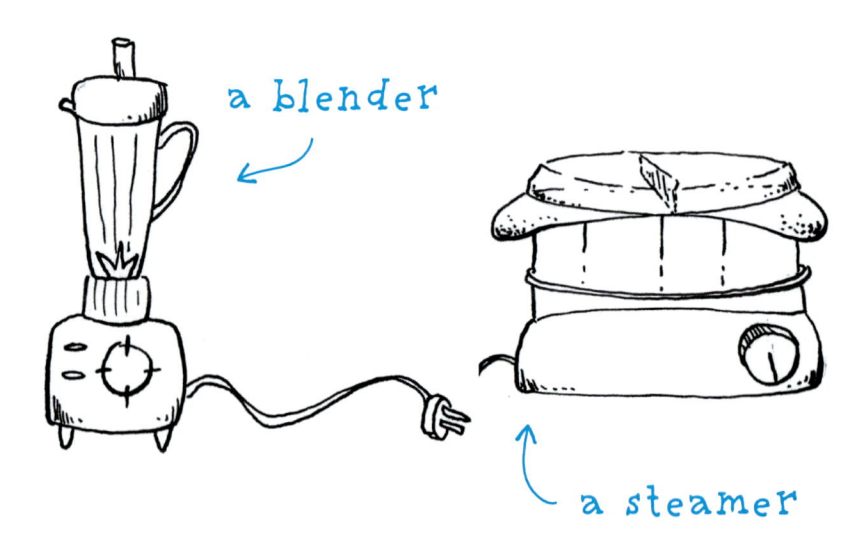

a blender

a steamer

- **a steamer.** This is inexpensive, easy to use, and particularly effective for people living on their own. It can even be installed in a corner of your room or dorm if you don't have easy access to a proper kitchen. A blender, steamer, and faucet are all you need to follow your 3-week Plan. I personally prefer electric appliances because their steam temperature is uniform. Choose the kind with a little tray that recovers the juices from the food you are steaming instead of mixing them with the boiling water. The best thing about an electric steamer is that it is 100 percent reliable. You don't need to be watching it while it does the job. You can do your 15-minute yoga workout, and dinner will be almost ready when you are done.

For your daily routine, you'll need:

- a yoga mat
- a tongue scraper
- massage oil. You can prepare this yourself by heating some sesame oil just to the point of boiling (test the temperature by adding a drop of water and turn off the heat when the water starts to fume). Then, add drops of your favorite essential oil (lavender, citrus, etc.).
- a harsh glove or a bath brush
- bath salts

Shopping time: Prepare a grocery list of all the "KEEP IN" ingredients that you think you are going to enjoy. If you have the budget and can go to a good natural store and a farmer's market, do so. Even though slightly more expensive, good produce is nutritionally dense, which means you'll buy less because you won't need as much food (and this will help your budget as well).

- You can buy all of these items at once: **dry produce,** such as nuts, seeds, nut and seed butters, rice, quinoa, **superfoods,** and frozen fruits and berries, if you have a freezer and are planning to use them. You may also buy your vegetable milks, oils, beans, and lentils. The best place to make these purchases is probably a health food store, although they are increasingly available in supermarkets lately. Carefully read through the ingredients, though. Not everything in a health food store is healthy!

- Have a look at the list of **recommended supplements** in the next chapter. Most of them can be purchased at the health food store as well.

- Also, look for things you are going to need for skin brushing, self massage, and bathing.

- Buy fresh produce twice a week to maximize its freshness. The best place for fresh produce is a farmer's market. Once you have found the most convenient one for you, it is nice to go back to the same person time and again to engage in conversation. You'll learn tons of information from these growers!

If you are in **college:**

- You may find some interesting ingredients for smoothies and lunches in the dining halls – go to the salad bar: choose raw foods and vegetables, lean proteins, and healthy fats.

- Buy the rest of the ingredients twice per week from the local grocery store.

- When at home, purchase supplements, superfoods, nuts, and seeds. These travel well, and your parents will be happy to see you taking an interest in "healthy things."

- Organize your dorm room kitchenette:
  * Some storage
  * A steamer and a personal blender
  * Your other utensils and dishware

Some buildings have community kitchen facilities. If yours doesn't, you can still make it work for one to two years in your dorm or studio apartment. You'll be a pro when you reach your own sweet little place!

Special note: It is probably easier if you schedule your 3-week Plan during some time at home. You will then know how to best care for yourself when you are back in college.

— plan your days —

- Find out how much time you are going to need in the morning in order to be able to do your yoga, skin brushing, oil massaging, and enjoying your nourishing, delicious breakfast. The whole thing shouldn't take you more than an hour.

- Think about where you're going to enjoy your lunch. Are you coming back home? Are you bringing your meal to your school or work place? Lunch is usually the easiest meal to eat at a restaurant or cafeteria but make careful choices and study the menu thoroughly.

- You want to try to avoid too many social events. 3 weeks without drinking can only do you good! You'll see that it is a good occasion to look inward and be calm.

CHAPTER 4

helpers

In this section, I am going to share some auxiliaries with you. These are actions and products other than foods that can help you succeed with the Plan. You're going to love these healthy daily habits!

hydration

Water is, of course, necessary for all the functions of your body. You already know that you are 70 percent water, and that adults lose, on average, three liters of fluid per day. Dehydration is probably the most common cause of digestive problems, lymph congestion, and poor detoxification function. Constant replenishment is essential and easily achieved by eating high-water-content foods or drinking eight glasses of water each day. But some of us, particularly during the winter months, don't feel like drinking all that water. Moreover, we have the impression that once we have forced ourselves into it, the water just passes through, and we need to run to empty our bladders.

I first heard about this rehydration technique from John Douillard, a doctor of Ayurvedic medicine. It is the best value-for-money treatment you can use…and it works for almost any ailment. People in the East use it all the time. It is inexpensive and requires nothing but water.

REHYDRATION TECHNIQUE

*"The best lymph moving re-hydration technique is to sip hot water every 10-15 minutes throughout the day.
Do it religiously for one day. If by the end of that day you are experiencing a dry mouth and are now thirsty for this once tasteless sip of hot water, this is a good indication you are dehydrated, and your lymph is congested.*

If this happens, try this re-hydration therapy: Sip Plain Hot Water (Boiled) every 10-15 min for five days. Boil the water that you want to drink for the day. You can carry a thermos with you to make it easy.

This is an ancient Ayurvedic method for flushing the lymphatic system, softening hardened tissues, and dilating, cleansing and then hydrating deep tissues. It also heals and repairs the digestive system and flushes the GALT (lymph on the outside of the intestinal wall)."

– Dr. Douillard at www.Lifespa.com

daily rituals

- Upon waking, start your day with a glass of hot water.

- You may then brush your teeth and scrape your tongue, removing any coating that will increasingly appear during the first days on the Plan but will then ease up.

- Yoga: try doing about 15 minutes of yoga every morning. It can be sun salutations, if you know how to do them. I usually do six rounds of sun salutations, followed by a couple of twists, an inverted pose, and five minutes of Pranayama. If you are not familiar with yoga or these poses, have a look on YouTube. You'll find an amazing new world.

- Finish your yoga routine with a few minutes of meditation (more on this in a later chapter).

- Before your daily shower, try dry brushing the skin of your entire body with a brush or a harsh glove. It shakes up your lymphatic system and alkalinizes your body.

- After the shower, apply the massage oil you made previously to your entire body and give yourself a five-minute self-massage.

- If you have access to a bath tub and have the time for indulging at the end of a tiring day, take a relaxing warm bath with alkalinizing salts. It's great for your mind, and it helps increase your body's alkalinity. A foot salt bath is another good (simpler) option.

elimination

You will probably start noticing a difference in your bowel movements from the rehydration and the early morning rituals. However, you want to be sure that you have a complete movement every single day that carries a maximum of toxins with it, the latest occurring after your breakfast. This can be very effectively enhanced with adequate fiber in your food. Fiber escorts toxic bile out of the intestines and into the toilet. Your now 'very high vegetable diet' is going to help you do that along with the right amount of chia seeds in your breakfast. Give it a try!

supplements

Following the advice of this new breed of doctors, who are better equipped to swing the pendulum toward prevention instead of focusing on treatment (I am talking about Functional Medicine, which addresses the underlying causes of disease), and particularly the wisdom of Dr. Perlmutter, I recommend that you take the following essential daily supplements during your 3-week Plan. Dr. Perlmutter recommends that you continue taking them for life!

- Coconut oil: One teaspoon daily, taken straight or used when preparing your meals.
- Probiotics: One capsule taken on an empty stomach (look for a probiotic that contains at least ten billion active cultures from at least ten different strains, including Lactobacillus acidophilus and Bifidobacterium). They help maintain a healthy inner ecology, improve digestion, increase immunity, and are cleansing.
- Vitamin D3: 5000IU daily
- Turmeric: 350mg twice daily. Combine this spice with black pepper for better results.
- DHA or fish oil capsules: 1000mg daily

CHAPTER 5

recipes and guides

At this point, you are probably thinking, "What am I actually going to eat?" And you surely are a little afraid of losing some of your favorite ingredients, not to mention snacks! But you'll see how straightforward and easy it gets with the guides and ideas I am about to share with you. Remember, this is an experiment, one on which you are going to build your new habits. So, go to your chopping boards, steamer, and/or blender and enjoy the ride!

breakfast guide and ideas

For the first meal of the day during the next 3 weeks, you are going to experiment with the following ingredients:

Fruit is a high-water-content food and a good fluid replenisher after the internal activity of the night's rest. There is a lot of literature on food combining and, in particular, fruit combining. I prefer to try things out and draw my own conclusions. Fruit alone, particularly if it is not rich in fiber, can provoke a glucose high in your blood, and we don't want that. To avoid this, try having some fat with it.

Nuts, seeds, nut and seed butters, and nut and seed milks. Not only are they going to provide the right healthy fat to keep sugar down and help you fast until lunch (two of their wonderful perks), but they are also rich in various minerals, which will help alkalinize your body.

Dark leafy greens are perfect foods that combine with everything and can (and should) be eaten at every meal.

Superfoods, of course!

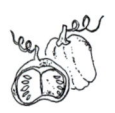

HOW ABOUT A SMOOTHIE?

A good blend of the following ingredients is a smoothie. This modern preparation has conquered the hearts of many. It is an easy to prepare, quick to take, versatile concoction of nourishing ingredients that work wonderfully for breakfast. Here is the guide for a perfect smoothie:

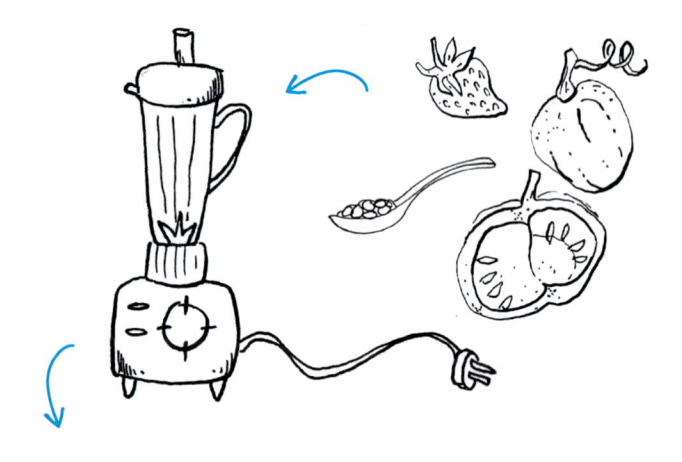

Choose one liquid and one or two fruits and/or vegetables. Blend in some nuts/seeds (nut/seed butters), one or several berries and/or greens. You may also add spices and/or superfoods. BLEND! Boosts and/or seeds may be added before or after blending depending on the texture you want to achieve. Always, always add some form of fat (nuts, seeds, avocado, coconut milk, etc.). Enjoy!

SMOOTHIE GUIDE	
Base (liquid)	Pure water Vegetable milks (grain/nut/seed): almond, hemp, hazelnut, quinoa, oat, rice, coconut Coconut water Chilled green or herbal tea Aloe vera juice
Fruits and vegetables	Apples, pears, bananas Berries: blueberries, raspberries, cherries, goji berries, cranberries (dried and frozen berries are an option) Mangoes, peaches, figs, apricots, prunes, kiwis, pineapples Cucumber, celery, pepper, beetroot
Nuts, seeds, and nut butters	Almonds, walnuts, hazelnuts, pine nuts, cashew nuts (use them raw and soak them overnight to improve digestion and enhance texture) Avocadoes, coconuts Chia seeds, flax seeds, hemp seeds, sunflower seeds, pumpkin seeds, linseeds Almond butter, sunflower seed butter, tahini, other nut/seed butters Coconut oil
Greens	Kale, spinach, romaine, arugula, celery stalks, dandelion greens, beet greens, parsley, cilantro, basil, mint
Spices	Cinnamon, nutmeg, vanilla, ginger, cayenne, turmeric, cardamom
Boosts/ superfoods	Cacao powder, maca powder, açai powder, goji berries, mulberries, dried cranberries, spirulina, chlorella

Some of **my favorite blends** are:

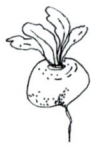

Apple, avocado, overnight soaked almonds (discard water), parsley, and rice milk. After blending, I add hemp seeds and goji berries on top.

Pear, celery stalk, overnight soaked walnuts (discard water), arugula, ginger, and aloe vera juice. I like to top this one with some more walnuts and dried mulberries.

Apple, overnight soaked almonds (discard water), overnight soaked dried apricots (use water), a cinnamon stick, and almond milk.

My **children's** favorites:

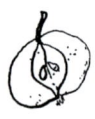

Apple, banana, almond butter, frozen raspberries, and rice milk. They don't much like having the superfoods on the top, so I sneak them in the mixture when they're not paying attention.

Mango, avocado, pear, and banana. A real sugar bomb! It is much too sweet for my taste, but they love it!

My **husband's** favorites:

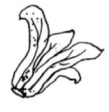

He loves vegetables in his, Vive la différence! Celery, cucumber, carrot, ginger, walnuts, and rice milk. He tops his with so many boosts and seeds that you can hardly see his smoothie at the bottom.

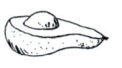

GET TO KNOW MOUSSE

Mousses are also wonderful. They are prepared with the same ingredients as smoothies but without the liquid.

Try an apple with overnight soaked hazelnuts (discard water) and soaked apricots (use water). Blend thoroughly until you achieve a smooth consistency. Add a cinnamon stick, and it will make you crazy for more!

Here's one my children love. Blend an avocado with lemon juice, a teaspoon of raw honey, and enough water to make it a "mousse." It is a delicious, rich cream that combines perfectly with fresh berries.

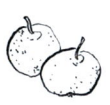

GRANOLA – ONLY BETTER

If you don't enjoy blended breakfasts, or if you feel like chewing or just don't have access to a blender, try using the same ingredients to prepare some sort of **fresh muesli.** Here are some nice ideas:

Grated apple and a sliced banana with almond butter, walnuts, raisins, Chia seeds, and goji berries. This is one of my favorites when fall arrives with its delicious apples and fresh walnuts!

Diced pear with hazelnut butter, pumpkin seeds, and shredded dry apricots, topped with hemp and chia seeds.

Sicilian oranges. You need to find top quality oranges for this one. Cut thin slices and distribute them on a plate in one layer, then drizzle with extra-virgin olive oil, and sprinkle with crumbled walnuts. Then, add sea salt flakes and a bit of cayenne. Incredible mixture!

lunch guide and ideas

In the middle of the day, your digestive strength is at its peak. Lunch should be the biggest meal of the day, and that's what you want to experiment with during the Plan. Here are the most suitable ingredients:

All kinds of vegetables. Put them in the center of your plate: raw, steamed, or sautéed. Use various types and colors and prepare them differently as well. Always include some green leaves, orange or red fruit-vegetables, something cooked, something raw, and a small portion of fermented vegetables and/or seaweed.

Choose an animal protein. Meat, fish, poultry, or eggs. When possible, choose wild, organic, or grazing animals. You may prepare these any way you want: marinated, steamed, sautéed with a bit of coconut or olive oil, or cooked in a casserole together with some vegetables. Canned fish is a suitable option when you need to pack your lunch but look for the cleanest options when shopping.

Or a vegetable protein. Beans, lentils, and chickpeas are all wonderful for lunch. They give a warm touch to salads and are very comforting in a stew in cold weather. They also transform wonderfully into hummus. Bloating might be a problem for you, but it will quite surely disappear if you soak/sprout them, cook them with a piece of Kombu seaweed, reduce the quantity per serving, or combine them well. They digest much better when combined with vegetables, leafy greens in particular. You may also use good quality cooked legumes, which are preserved in glass jars. Remember to select those that just have water or a little salt added.
It is so easy to prepare lunch using legumes!

Or grains. Rice (choose whole rice, real Italian risotto, or Spanish paella rice), quinoa, amaranth, millet, and buckwheat. They all work great at lunch when combined with vegetables, and they can be prepared in advance. For instance, during the weekend, prepare two or three servings. Then, during the week, they will be ready and waiting for you to add some raw and cooked vegetables, olives, aromatic herbs, etc. for an easy-to-make-and-take lunch.

Fat. Absolutely indispensable at every meal. You can use it for cooking. Choose coconut, sesame, or olive oil. I know there is a lot of confusion over whether to heat the olive oil or not. When I am concerned about toxicity, I like to look at epidemiology, and I have learned that olive oil has been used for cooking in Mediterranean countries for centuries without ever being the source of health problems. Unsweetened coconut cream or milk is something you may want to consider, too. It gives just the right touch when preparing curried vegetables. And then, of course, olives, nuts, seeds, and avocados. You can never have too many avocados. The quantity of avocados I consume is ridiculous!

Most people cannot leave the table at lunch without having a little sweet. If this is the case for you, your best option is one square of very dark chocolate (I am talking about 80% or more) that you can savor by enjoying it with 4–5 hazelnuts. A mixture of raw honey and tahini, a sesame seed butter widely used in the Middle East, is also delicious. Greeks even have a name for that. They call it Halva.

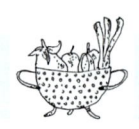

VEGETARIAN MIXES

Indian. Dice 4–5 different vegetables, such as sweet potato, zucchini, carrot, pepper, eggplant, etc. and steam them for 10 minutes. In a saucepan, melt some coconut oil and roast a diced garlic clove and some cumin, then add the steamed vegetables. On low heat, add turmeric and black pepper or a good curry blend. You can then add a cup of coconut milk and salt, and cook it just long enough for the flavors to mingle. Top it with abundant coriander and cayenne pepper. You may want to combine this with rice or another grain of your choice.

Peruvian. Use about a cup of previously cooked quinoa as a base, and then add an abundant mixture of raw greens (parsley, coriander, mint, basil, etc.), some diced green peppers, and black olives. Season with salt and sprinkle with a generous quantity of olive oil. Cayenne on the top is optional.

Korean. Use about a cup of previously cooked whole rice. In a saucepan, heat some sesame oil, then add two cloves of sliced garlic and one shiitake mushroom. On medium heat, add some nice greens (Swiss chard, broccolini, spinach, collard greens, etc.), put the lid on, and allow them to cook slightly for five minutes. Then deglaze with some tamari, mix in the rice, and sprinkle with black sesame seeds.

Italian. You may also want to use the technique above to prepare a simple risotto. Start by sautéing something nice in the saucepan with olive oil, onion, and/or garlic: it can be zucchini, fennel, beetroot, pumpkin, peppers, any kind of mushrooms, or any greens. Then add the pre-cooked rice and finish by adding flavor from a lemon rind, cayenne pepper, basil, or brewer's yeast (similar to nutritional yeast), which will give it a cheesy flavor.

Spanish. In the summer in Spain, we prepare a great deal of bean, chickpea, and lentil salads. We cook the beans in advance, making sure that they are a little crunchy. You can do this or use a jar of organic precooked legumes. Then add as many colorful raw summer vegetables as you have in your fridge: yellow, green, and red peppers, cucumber, fennel, or white onions. Then add a sizable quantity of olive oil, capers, and olives, and you can finish it off by adding parsley, coriander, and/or basil. A touch of raw garlic is most welcome in this recipe if you like it.

— using animal protein —

Top quality eggs, fish, and meat don't need complicated recipes. You just need a little imagination and a lot of vegetables. Everyone knows how to cook an omelet with veggies and how to add hard-boiled eggs to a colorful salad. You can even go Japanese-style and enjoy a lightly steamed egg over miso soup, which you can have as a starter before some stir-fried vegetables.

For fish, the steamer is extremely useful. You can either cook it by itself and then crumble it onto your mixed vegetables or cook it together with the vegetables in a little wax paper packet in your steamer.

I am not a meat eater myself, but I cook it for the family. I obtain the best results when I marinate it with herbs and tamari and then cook it in the oven at a very low temperature. After it is cooked, you can keep it in your fridge and slice it over vegetables when preparing your lunch. Always freshen up leftovers by adding aromatic herbs, cayenne pepper, a dash of olive oil, and some tamari.

dinner guide and ideas

At the end of the day, the sun is setting, and it has probably all but disappeared before you have the opportunity to start thinking about dinner. Overall energy is low, and you want to go with the flow in this 3-week Plan, so a lighter meal is ideal at this time of the day. One that's going to be — you guessed it — full of vegetables. The easiest option for a light dinner rich in vegetables is, of course, soup. If you want to give it a try, have a look at the soup guide below:

SOUP GUIDE	
Root vegetables	Potato, carrot, sweet potato, leek, onion, garlic…
Fruit vegetables	Zucchini, eggplant, tomato, peppers, pumpkin, green beans…
Flower vegetables	Cauliflower, broccoli, cabbage…
Leafy greens	Kale, spinach, romaine, arugula, dandelion greens, beet greens, parsley, cilantro, basil, mint…
Legumes	Beans, lentils, chickpeas…
Seaweed	Dulse, arame, hijiki…
Oils	Cold-pressed olive oil, coconut oil, and coconut cream
Spices	Sea salt, tamari, oregano, curcuma, cumin, nutmeg, pepper…

EASY STEAMED VEGETABLE SOUP

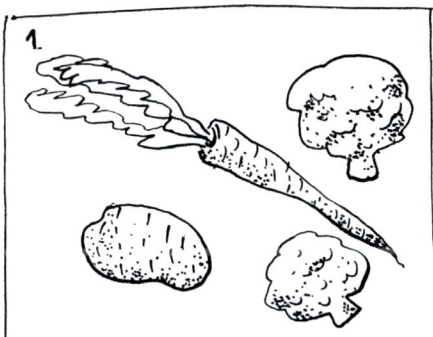

1. Choose a minimum of 3 vegetables. Wash them and peel when necessary. Cut them into chunks.

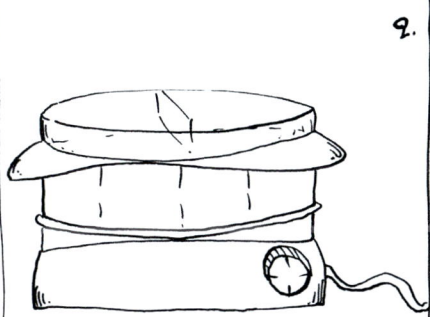

2. Put them into your steamer's basket and cook for 20 min.

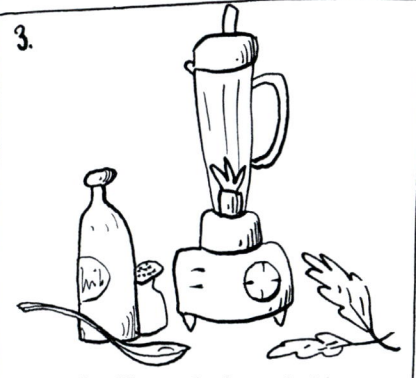

3. Transfer the cooked vegetables plus the cooking juices to your blender. Add olive or coconut oil, sea salt or tamari, plus herbs, leafy greens and/or spices. Blend!

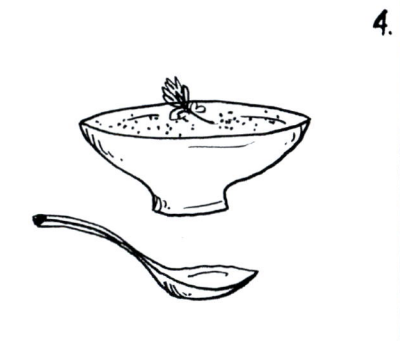

4. Serve: it's ready!

Choose a minimum of three vegetables that'll blend harmoniously in taste and color. You can either steam or boil your vegetables. Legumes need to be either sprouted and then steamed or boiled, or soaked and cooked separately. In warm weather, you can prepare a completely raw soup. Most leafy greens can (and should) be eaten raw. So add those after cooking, together with oil, spices, seaweed, and some boiling water (if needed) to achieve the right consistency. BLEND! Enjoy!

Fresh soup is really easy to cook, so try preparing a new one each day. You'll feel the difference!

I prepare my soups in the steamer and then play with spices, herbs, oils, and different consistencies to create an interesting new preparation every evening.

These are **client and fan favorites:**

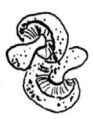

Place pumpkin, red pepper, and one garlic clove in the steamer for 20 minutes. Then blend into a thin unctuous cream with coconut milk, cumin, turmeric, lemongrass, and tamari.

Cook leeks and zucchini in the steamer for 15 minutes. Blend with baby spinach, olive oil, sea salt, and some boiling water, if needed. The almost phosphorescent green color that you achieve by adding young leafy greens to your blends is mind-blowing! This one also works very well with some broccoli.

Instant minestrone: steam diced red pepper, eggplant, carrot, potato, tomato, and leeks for 20 minutes. Then blend very lightly, in order to keep a coarse texture, with olive oil, lemon rind, and oregano. Add salt to taste. You may also want to add freshly prepared pesto to this one, which you can get by blending a little handful of pine nuts or raw almonds, basil leaves, olive oil, and salt.

Gazpacho is just for the summer or very warm areas. Not only because you drink it cold but even more so because you need to prepare it with the nicest tomatoes that you can find. Blend as many tomatoes as you can eat in one serving with half a cucumber, a light green Italian pepper (green bell peppers are also good if you cannot find these), sea salt, plenty of olive oil, and apple cider vinegar. Then add some ice cubes and blend again.

> Raw avocado soup. Even if it is all raw, this one is much warmer than gazpacho. Blend one avocado with the juice of one lemon, a little garlic clove (optional), baby spinach and/or cilantro, olive oil, tamari, and enough water to achieve a nice creamy consistency.

The combinations are endless, and you are going to find, as I did, that steamed soup is a very versatile, affordable (both money and difficulty-wise), quick way to have a nice wholesome dinner. You may want to add legumes if you feel you need more nutrition, or you may even want to include some of your superfoods. You can keep it light if your goal is to lose weight. This is actually the only meal that you want to keep light when trying to reduce your waistline. It can take a little longer than with harsh diets, but the weight will stay off! And believe me, preconceptions aside, there is nothing boring about fresh vegetable soups like the ones I've just described.

You can also have all the above ingredients and **combinations** in the form of salads, stews, stir-fries, and even steamed and tossed with homemade vinaigrette (made from olive oil, lemon, shallots and/or lemon rind, and salt).

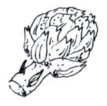

> Avocado (once again!) with tomatoes, white onions, olives, arugula, plenty of olive oil, lemon juice, and salt is yummy! You can have this at lunch as well by adding some canned fish.
>
> Potato salad is also great in the evening. Steam some firm sliced potatoes for 20 minutes. In the last 10 minutes, add a handful of string beans. When they are done cooking, place them in a bowl with diced tomatoes, sliced red onion, black olives, capers, parsley, coriander, sea salt, and plenty of olive oil.

Use the above guides and ideas as a canvas, and, for 3 weeks, plunge into this intuitive and creative approach. It's time to experiment! This is when your journal is going to come in handy. Record what you liked and disliked (that brownish yucky smoothie!), and even more important, write about how these new preparations made you feel.

If you need more inspiration, real recipes, and pictures, you can go to my website: www.teresafernandez-gil.com.

two more tips

There are two more things that are of great importance when it comes to the act of eating. One is **saying grace.** Once your dish is ready, take some time to acknowledge all of the effort it has taken for that food to arrive in front of you. Honor the food you buy and the food you cook as you would the food that you grow. You can do it in a religious way or some other way. At home, we like to change the formula to increase awareness, but one version that will stay in the memories of my children forever is, "Let's eat with love what has been produced with love, prepared with love, and served with love."

The other important thing, more down to Earth, is **chewing**. You may have already heard that digestion begins with the chewing process. If you skip the salivation and trituration stage (this literally means pulverizing the food by chewing it thoroughly), your food is more likely to ferment in your bowels, provoking bloating and tiredness. Bringing the mindfulness you just created by saying grace into the process of chewing will offer you that blissful moment of conscious eating that is so rewarding for both your body and your soul.

CHAPTER 6

wrapping up at the end of the 3 weeks

21 days is a well-documented expanse of time in which new habits become routine. When you want your boyfriend, girlfriend, roommate, etc. to take on some new chore, just say, "Do it for just 3 weeks, and then I'll do it." Apparently, after 21 days, they'll continue on without even noticing. So, that's the purpose of this program. Provided that you are feeling good when you finish it, your body is going to ask you to go on in one way or another.

so what happens after the Plan?

The testing week is the last stage of the program. The purpose of it is to identify your very own disruptors and to dwell even deeper into your bio-individuality. One of the reasons you feel good at the end of the 3 weeks is because you have removed the most common pro-inflammatory foods and toxic triggers and given your digestive and immune system some rest. The goal now is to try to evaluate those irritants by following a testing period.

test one food for one day at all three meals

Gluten and dairy are among the most common groups of disturbing foods, but you may use this technique with other foods or food groups that you suspect can be problematic for you. Choose one (and only one) of the foods or food groups you want to test and use it at every meal for one whole day. Do this on the day after you finish the 3-week Plan. You may do this for any specific food item that you want to check. For instance, soy, eggs, or corn. Don't try alcohol at every meal, though! You already know its effects! The goal is to isolate your body's reaction to a specific food. Record your reactions and feelings in your journal, including how you feel right after eating, your energy levels in the following hours, bowel movements, and changes in sleep and/or emotions.

If you have a strong negative reaction, this is your body's way of telling you to eliminate this food from your diet completely for a period of time. Quite often, after a periodic regeneration of your digestive system, you will see that yesterday's difficult to digest foods can be welcomed back into your diet. If your reaction is mild, my advice is to give it a try from time to time and act accordingly.

what happens next?

There are two scenarios:

- **"I feel great!"** After the 3-week Plan, you feel great, enjoy the recipes, love your daily routine, and want to continue. Why not? There is no reason not to maintain this lifestyle. You'll get healthier, lighter, and happier every day!

- **"I feel good but I need to relax a little"** or, **"I'm not ready to maintain this approach 100%."** You feel good, but the Plan didn't seem to reveal any clear disruptors for you, and, moreover, you want to move on to a more social life.
I suggest you keep some of the elements that worked best for you: smoothies, three meals per day, no snacks, morning routine, chewing, food combining, etc. and try the Plan once more when your body asks for it. In the meantime, be flexible but mindful. The rules are not there to make you agonize over them. Don't be a bore to yourself or others. Do things from your heart because what you feel deep inside is right. Every day is a conversation between you and your body.

EXTRA ADVICE

other cares of the self

Lately, I have been more and more interested in ancient health traditions. More holistic than our Western medicine, they view health as more than the absence of disease. I have followed Traditional Chinese Medicine and Ayurveda in the works of Paul Pitchford, Deepak Chopra, and John Douillard, whom I find particularly inspiring. Although I am far from being an expert, I have introduced, both in my life and the practice of my profession, some simple techniques that have proven to be terribly useful. I have already shared some with you, like the rehydration technique. I'd like to briefly enumerate a few others that can help you in your quest for balance.

— yoga —

It's a complete exercise that simultaneously integrates one's whole physiology: mind, body, and breath. It strengthens and stretches all the major muscle groups, lubricates the joints, flexes the spine, and massages the internal organs. Blood flow and circulation are increased throughout the body, and with regular practice, you will gain stability, suppleness, flexibility, and grace. If you are new to Yoga, I suggest that you start with an instructor. It has taken me close to twenty years to have a self-guided practice!

— breathing techniques and mindfulness —

Breathing is the basic rhythm of life that supports all other rhythms. Many Ayurvedic routines help to bring breathing back into balance. As an introduction to this practice, I recommend Dr. Douillard's One-Minute Meditation:

ONE-MINUTE MEDITATION

"Sit in a comfortable position, in a chair with a straight back or on the floor in a cross-legged position. Breathe deeply in and out through the nose for 30 breaths, which is roughly 30 seconds, or one breath in and out per second. Try to fill the lungs as deeply as you can and empty them as completely as you can on the exhale. While the priority is breathing as deeply as possible, you are also trying to breathe in and out at a rapid, but comfortable rhythmic pace. It is a fast, deep, but comfortable pumping breath through the nose, hence the name, Bellows Breath. When you complete the Bellows Breaths, just sit still with your eyes closed for 30 seconds, experiencing the qualities of this stillness. After 30 seconds, slowly open your eyes and notice if you feel calmer with fewer thoughts. Then, carry this calm into your activity and notice the difference. Over time, you will become aware of when you start to lose that heightened sense of centeredness and awareness, at which point you should do the One Minute Meditation again. When you do this 5–10 times a day, you slowly build a reservoir of oxygen and Prana in the blood and brain that begins to assure the brain that it is safe to be calm, safe to be relaxed, and safe to carry this calm into everyday activities."

– Dr. Douillard at www.Lifespa.com

This can be the first step in your journey to a successful and transformational meditation (mindfulness) practice.

―――――――――――

"Meditation is not forcing yourself to be quiet. It is finding the quiet that is already there."
– Deepak Chopra

―――――――――――

— exercising —

Charaka, the greatest writer on Ayurveda, gives this very complete explanation for the need for exercise:

―――――――――――

"From physical exercise one gets lightness, a capacity for work, firmness, tolerance of difficulties, elimination of impurities, and stimulation of digestion."
– Charaka

―――――――――――

The ideal exercise is one that balances the whole system. Walking and cycling are both pretty ideal exercises that should be integrated as much as possible into your daily routines. I also love to recommend Dr. Douillard's 12-minute workout, as he says "less is more."

12-MINUTE WORKOUT

"Go for a walk, jog, bike ride or use a cardio machine like an elliptical trainer. Step One: Warm up Exercise slowly for 2 minutes while maximally breathing in and out through your nose. Nasal breathing is a skill that may take some time to master. Do the best you can and, in time, the nasal breathing will get easier. Step Two: Sprint Start exercising faster, like a mini sprint for 1 minute. Use the nasal breath during the sprint if you can as it will slow you down and not let you do too much. Don't push it here. Start slow and build yourself up to a faster sprint over time. Try to do a sprint pace that you can maintain for one minute. In a couple of weeks, you will be sprinting like a pro. Step 3: Recovery Slow the exercise down to the Warm Up pace for one minute and maintain the nasal breathing if you can. Nasal Breathing during the recovery will force air into the lower lobes of the lungs allowing for more efficient release of CO_2 and activation of the calming parasympathetic nervous system that predominates in the lower lobes of the lungs. This will help you release toxins and stress. Step 4: Second Sprint Start another sprint for one minute. Make this a little faster if you can. Continue nasal breathing if possible. Sprints can be running up and down stairs, jumping jacks, jumping on and off a curb for one minute, just get the exertion level up. Step 5: Second Recovery Recover from the sprint with one minute of deep nasal breathing at the warm up pace. If you cannot maintain nasal breathing during the recovery, the sprint was too hard. Each time it will get easier. Step 6: Continue Sprints and Recoveries for a total of 3 sprints and 3 recoveries. Follow the nasal breathing if you can.

– Dr. Douillard at www.Lifespa.com

While the fitness benefits of exercise are undeniable, it is important to reduce the amount of stress that is perceived by the body during a workout and the domino effect of hormonal responses that follow. As it turns out, how you breathe determines how you respond to stress. When we breathe through our noses, the incoming air is forced through the nose deeply into the lower lobes of the lungs where the calming, repairing parasympathetic nerve receptors predominate. In other words, breathing through the nose during exercise is a tool that can alter the body's perception of the activity it normally perceives as stressful, to one of calm and repair.

This 12-minute routine can be performed daily or a minimum of three times per week. You can use this as your entire workout or as a cardiovascular warm up before yoga, bike riding, or hiking. I personally enjoy doing this with a skipping rope. In this way, I can exercise wherever and whenever I want, even when travelling, with a minimum of paraphernalia…and at no cost.
Oh are you going to love your body after starting this routine!

— sleeping —

*"We are meant to ride nature's waves,
not to fight against them."*
– Deepak Chopra

One of the most basic aspects of living in tune with nature is to respect its cycles. The only way to achieve this is by maintaining regular sleep habits. This means going to bed and waking up more or less at the same hours throughout the week, even throughout the year, with little seasonal variations. A consistent bedtime routine helps. Do whatever you need to do to wind down and tell your body that it is time to go to sleep. Caffeine, alcohol, and nicotine aren't good sleep companions. An early dinner, a calm stroll, deep breathing, meditation, and massaging your feet with warm oil are. If you do all of this at the end of one of your Plan days, you will probably sleep like a hibernating bear!

— being in nature —

Most people, and very particularly those living in large cities, have a clear vitamin N deficit disorder, where N stands for Nature. Every week, schedule some time to take advantage of Nature's gifts: walk barefoot through the grass or on a beach, sunbathe naked, take a walk in the woods or beside the ocean, a lake, or a stream, listen to the birds, and watch the stars.

"Nature provides a rich source of energy and nourishment that has healing effects on both body and mind."
– Deepak Chopra

other useful concepts

Primary food. This interesting concept is one of the pillars in the teaching at the IIN® School (Institute for Integrative Nutrition), where I completed the last stretch of my studies. For me, it has added a lot of sense to my professional practice. Primary food is what feeds you (without being on your plate): healthy relationships, regular physical activity, a fulfilling career, and a spiritual practice. All these elements are essential forms of nourishment. When we use real (secondary) food as a way to alleviate or suppress our hunger for primary food, the body and mind suffer.

Vegetarianism. More and more people think that eating animal products is a question of ethics. A vegan lifestyle (not eating any food from animal sources, even honey) is increasingly popular among the young. From the environmental point of view, it would be ideal if we all become vegetarians or vegans. But many people feel very strongly about their need to eat animal flesh and products in order to be healthy. Vegetarians and vegans extract most of their protein from beans, which is quite challenging because even if beans are perfectly healthy, they are among the most difficult foods to digest. This 3-week Plan is an opportunity to experiment with food in a way that can help you find balance in your individual needs for different kinds of protein.

Sustainability. When thinking about food and health, we can no longer reduce it to our own physical health. It is not possible to separate the health of our body from that of the environment. Everything is linked, and we must consider the health of all things: the soil, plants, animals, and ourselves. When you eat a natural, seasonal, local, and fresh diet rich in plants, you will help to make life on our planet more sustainable. There is a clear cry out there for real sustainable food. You can't possibly have missed the frequent articles in blogs and newspapers about meat and the carbon footprint, overfishing, the rebirth of farmer's markets, and a new movement called "rural by choice." So, even if big Agro wants its profits, at the end of the day, it is you, the consumer, who commands. In the words of Michael Pollan, "We are entering a postindustrial era of food."

when out of track

Most of this book focuses on helping you build a more balanced, happier, and overall healthier life. And you definitely will if you follow these instructions. Most minor ailments are also going to become rare.

The first thing you will notice when you are in tune is the beautiful complexion of your skin, so when **skin impurities** come back ... you know what you have to do. Another great benefit of this way of eating is an enhanced body shape, particularly the disappearance of your **belly fat.** So if you see it resurfacing, that is another sign that you need to check back. The 3–meal-a-day Plan is a sure way to control most stress, particularly if you couple it with the breathing techniques. Meditation and breathing techniques are also extremely useful when fighting against **addictions.** And, believe it or not, most cases of **depression** are also healed by a good food routine based on three meals a day that are rich in top quality protein and fat. Julia Ross, the author of an interesting book called, The Mood Cure, says "Junk moods come from junk foods." High glycemic index foods and lack of sufficient healthy fat and protein have been proven to be powerful factors in brain degeneration and cognitive impairment, including depression.

Ladies only: The balance of female hormones in a woman's body is important for optimal health, including cancer prevention. The best way to assess your hormonal balance is by closely watching your cycle. Most common symptoms of hormonal imbalance are due to excessive estrogen: PCOS, fibroids, ovarian cysts, infertility, and low libido. These, and most hormonal imbalances, can be traced back to a lymphatic traffic jam! These are the symptoms: pain, irregular periods, overly heavy periods, missing periods, breast tenderness, bloating, water retention, and skin breakouts. The quality, duration, comfort level, and timing of your menses offer a monthly opportunity to evaluate your lymphatic function. Always try lymphatic (non- intrusive) therapies before hormonal ones. You know them: alkalinize your diet, rehydrate, brush and self-massage your skin, and reduce stressors.

Voilà! You now have all of the necessary tools to achieve a balanced young adult life. So, if once in a while you are tempted to overindulge by **"living la vida loca,"** just go back to page one and follow the 3-week Plan again!
You can also reach me at www.teresafernandez-gil.com.

favorite reading list

Body, Mind and Sport: the Mind-Body Guide to life-long Health, Fitness and your Personal Best by John Douillard (Harmony Books, 1994)

Clean: The Revolutionary Program to Restore the Body's Natural Ability to Heal Itself by Alejandro Junger, MD (HarperOne, Second Updated Edition, 2012)

Conscious Eating by Gabriel Cousens, MD (North Atlantic Books, Second Edition, 2000)

Diet for a New America by John Robbins (HJ Kramer/New World Library, 25th Anniversary Edition, 2012)

Food Matters: A Guide to Conscious Eating by Mark Bittman (Simon & Schuster, 2009)

Food Rules: An Eater's Manual by Michael Pollan (Penguin Books, 2009)

Grain Brain: The Surprising Truth about Wheat, Carbs, and Sugar – Your Brain's Silent Killers by David Perlmutter, MD (Little, Brown, and Company, 2013)

Healing with Whole Foods: Asian Traditions and Modern Nutrition by Paul Pitchford (North Atlantic Books, Third Revised Expanded Edition, 2002)

In Defense of Food: An Eater's Manifesto by Michael Pollan (Penguin Books, 2009)

Integrative Nutrition: Feed Your Hunger for Health & Happiness by Joshua Rosenthal (Integrative Nutrition Pub., Third Edition, 2014)

Light on life. The Yoga Journey to Wholeness, Inner Peace, and Ultimate Freedom by B. K. S. Iyengar (Rodale, 2005)

Nutrition and Physical Degeneration by Weston A. Price (Benediction Classics, 2010)

Perfect Health: the Complete Mind Body Guide by Deepak Chopra (Three Rivers Press, 2000)

The Blender Girl: 100 gluten-free, vegan recipes by Tess Masters (Ten Speed Press, 2014)

The China Study: The Most Comprehensive Study of Nutrition Ever Conducted and the Startling Implications for Diet, Weight-Loss, and Long Term Health by T. Collin Campbell and Thomas M. Campbell II (BenaBella Books, 2006)

The Hippocrates Diet and Health Program by Anne Wigmore (Avery Trade, 1983)

The Mood Cure: Take Charge of Your Emotions in 24 Hours Using Food and Supplements by Julia Ross (Thorsons, 2003)

favorite websites

Dr. Alejandro Junger – www.cleanprogram.com

Dr. Andrew Weil – www.drweil.com

Dr. Frank Lipman – www.drfranklipman.com

Dr. John Douillard – www.lifespa.com

Dr. Mark Hyman – www.drhyman.com

www.Integrativenutrition.com

Julia Ross – www.themoodcure.com

www.Nutritionstripped.com

acknowledgements

It takes so much to complete what seems like a little project...such as this one: so many discussions, encounters, and inspirations, as well as extensive help and guidance. I want to start by acknowledging my deep gratitude for my children: Alvaro, Pedro, Clara, and Ana Teresa – you are the inspiration for this book. Many thanks go to José, who still believes in, and supports, my many, ever-changing projects. Thank you Joshua Rosenthal and Lindsay Smith from the Institute for Integrative Nutrition for your fabulous Launch A Book Program. Much heartfelt gratitude to Kathy, who has been there through the whole process. And to Georgina who pushed me at the right time. Thanks to Joanna and Karen, who put me on the right track for writing in English. Again, thanks to Alvaro and Pedro, my pre-proofreaders. And to Tracy, my editor – what a great discovery! She has given my work the touch of an angel. Thank you, Leila – your cover drawing is the final touch that I needed. Thank you, Florence, for shaping the project so nicely. And, of course, I thank my family and friends who have endured hours and hours of nutrition discussions and experimenting. I feel very grateful to the many teachers I have encountered in this never-ending quest on human nutrition; their amazing work inspires me every day.